Happy Calories Don't Count!

(neither does unhappy exercise)

Happy Calories Don't Count!
(neither does unhappy exercise)

Carmela Ramaglia

A division of
POWER WITHIN PRODUCTIONS, INC.
SEATTLE, WA

Copyright © 2010 by Carmela Ramaglia

Published by Power Within Publishing
A division of Power Within Productions, Inc.
www.powerwithinpublishing.com

Cover Photography: Marc Von Borstel

All rights reserved. This book may not be reproduced in whole or in part without written permission from the publisher, except by a reviewer, who may quote brief passages in a review; nor may any part of this book be reproduced, stored in a retrieval system, or transmitted in any form or by any means, electronic, mechanical, photocopying, or other, without written permission from the publisher. The intent of the author is only to offer information of a general nature to help you in your quest for physical, emotional and spiritual well-being. In the event you use any of the information in this book for yourself, which is your constitutional right, the author and the publisher assume no responsibility for your actions. Although it is difficult to know the original author of many sayings, adages, affirmations, and quotes, every effort is made to give credit to the most recent source. The author and publisher do not suggest any affiliation or association with any individual mentioned.

Library of Congress Control Number: 2010935117

ISBN 978-0-9828656-0-6
Printed in the United States on acid- free paper
Distributed by Power Within Publishing

FOR MOM

for loving me through thin and thick

Contents

1.
The School of Hard Knocks   1

2.
There are no "Once and for All
– Forever and All Time" Solutions   15

3.
Happy Happy – Joy Joy   29

4.
Let's Get Physical   37

5.
Let's Get Meta-Physical   47

6.
Tools of the Trade   55

7.
Repeat After Me: "All Is Well in My World"   65

8.
The Fifth Element   77

9.
The Body Shop   83

10.
In Other Words   93

Acknowledgements

I'D LIKE TO THANK EVERY CALORIE I'VE EVER CONSUMED (or haven't) and every calorie I've ever burned (or haven't). Thank you to Joshie for encouraging me to write about all those calories. Thanks to Pops for teaching me about the "school of hard knocks." You were right – there really is a "devil" in the mirror. Thank you to Sister for being the only one who truly understands and for making me watch *The Fifth Element*. Finally, thank you to Poochie for always making me happy.

I'd also like to thank all of my Pilates instructors, Rolfers, Hellerworkers and clients. You've taught me so much! And a very special thank you to Marianne Williamson and to Louise Hay, whose work helped me when I needed it the most.

Acknowledgements

I'D LIKE TO THANK EVERY CALORIE I'VE EVER CONSUMED (or haven't) and every calorie I've ever burned (or haven't). Thank you to Joshie for encouraging me to write about all those calories. Thanks to Pops for teaching me about the "school of hard knocks." You were right – there really is a "devil" in the mirror. Thank you to Sister for being the only one who truly understands and for making me watch *The Fifth Element*. Finally, thank you to Poochie for always making me happy.

I'd also like to thank all of my Pilates instructors, Rolfers, Hellerworkers and clients. You've taught me so much! And a very special thank you to Marianne Williamson and to Louise Hay, whose work helped me when I needed it the most.

Be patient toward all that is unsolved in your heart.
Try to love the questions themselves.
Do not now seek the answers which cannot be given
because you would not be able to live them.
And the point is to live everything.
Live the questions now.
Perhaps you will then gradually,
without noticing it,
Live along some distant day
into the answers.

― Rainer Maria Rilke

And then the day came
when the risk to remain tight inside the bud
was more painful than the risk it took to blossom.

- Anaïs Nin

1

The School of Hard Knocks

I HAVE LEARNED THAT IT'S ALL ABOUT BEING HAPPY. The only reason we ever want anything is because we think that having it will make us happy. It's a fundamental, universal truth and to understand the power of this concept I accidentally put into practice, it helps to know a little bit about the perspective from which I come.

When I was fifteen I made the varsity cheerleading squad. After our uniform fitting I decided to go on a diet. I knew how short those skirts were going to be and I wanted to look good. It was no big deal; I simply cut out everything I considered "junk food" – no cookies, candy, chips, etc. If it had "no nutritional value" in my mind, I didn't eat it. I wasn't very sophisticated in reading food labels back then, so I still ate plenty of things like high-sugar, full-fat yogurt and those oversized honey-bran muffins, thinking they were "good for me." I did lose weight over the summer. I don't remember how much, but it was enough to get plenty of "oh my gosh – you look so good!" comments from all the girls – and boys – at school. Somewhere along the line, I don't know when or how, my little "no junk food" diet turned into full-blown anorexia.

Eating disorders are big, complicated messes full of emotional, psychological and oftentimes, familial issues. There are plenty of memoirs and other books detailing the horrors of eating disorders. For me, it's simply part of the story, something that needs to be mentioned so you can understand the message I'm trying to impart.

I spent the summer between my junior and senior years of high school exercising, literally. I was following a basic "calories out more than calories in equals weight loss" approach to my body. I was exercising six to eight hours a day (it was summer and I had nothing better to do) and subsisting on barely 500 calories a day, spread over three meager meals.

I don't really remember my senior year of high school. I spent most of it in the hospital, where they tried to "cure" me by making me eat and by filling my days with therapy. Needless to say, the hospital's "calories in more than calories out equals weight gain" approach was working and I wasn't very happy about it.

College was a very difficult and scary time for me. It is ironic because now I look back on my undergraduate days as some of the best in my life. I knew how to lose weight – I was very good at it. And I knew how to gain weight – the hospital made me do that. But I didn't know how to maintain my weight. I didn't know that magic combination of "calories in equal calories out equals maintaining weight." I was terrified of eating too much and gaining weight, yet I was also terrified of not eating enough, losing weight and ending up back in the hospital. Somehow I managed to navigate the structure of my class schedule and the three meals a day provided by the student cafeteria and make it all work.

After graduation, though, my life fell apart. Suddenly I was forced to live in the "real world" and have a job. My undergraduate degree is in economics and while many of my friends were working for big firms, I couldn't bear the thought of sitting at a desk eight hours a day – think of all the weight I would gain! So instead, I opted for retail and serving positions where I could stand up and walk around all day.

The School of Hard Knocks

At twenty-two, my first nervous breakdown was quickly approaching. I was gaining weight and I didn't know why. I was exercising more and more (getting up at 4:30 in the morning to get in those two hours before work) and eating less and less and I was *gaining* weight! I went to a doctor about it; she thought I was crazy and sent me to therapy. After a few months of therapy I couldn't take it anymore. I cashed out my savings and checked out of the real world. I went to Italy, where I spent the summer walking the hills of Tuscany, not eating and losing 30 pounds.

Full of resolve that I would never have to deal with this again, I spent the next year monitoring my food and exercise very carefully. Yet it wasn't working – I still gained weight. This time the doctors said that I had "messed up my metabolism" by being anorexic. Well, I couldn't deal with that, so I took every last penny I had and headed back to Italy. Unable to bear the record-breaking summer heat, I packed up and headed north to cooler Paris. I took long walks along the Seine, ate very little and didn't lose a pound.

I came home and ended up in the hospital yet again. I didn't know then that those 30 painful pounds I had been obsessing over were nothing. At my heaviest I was still only 120 pounds, and my entire world was about to come crashing down around me.

Almost immediately after being released from the hospital, I got involved with a body builder (yes, I know). But this guy owned a gym and if I dated him it would be impossible not to lose weight and get the body I wanted, right? Needless to say, it did not work out. Not only did it not work out, I ended up another 25 pounds heavier.

I needed an escape. I'd already done the Europe thing – twice – and had no savings left to speak of. What would I do now? Graduate school! I took out a huge student loan (which I am still paying off) and ran away. While I was in school I found an "expert," followed a specific food and exercise program, and I lost weight.

Life is a funny thing, though. By the middle of my graduate program I had finally "conquered" my food dilemmas. I found a diet and exercise program that worked. I was in the best shape of my life and feeling good about it. But I hadn't quite dealt with all the emotional and psychological garbage that comes along with eating disorders and one not-so-tiny emotional setback turned my controlled eating and exercise into compulsive overeating and no exercise.

I finished my graduate program at nearly 200 pounds. I was lost. I was broken. I tried to pick up the pieces again – I really did. I hit the gym (which felt very uncomfortable in that body) and I went on a myriad of diets. I read nearly every book published on weight loss at the time and went back into therapy. I tried personal trainers. I tried nutritionists. I tried supplements. I tried acupuncture. I tried hypnosis. I tried affirmations. I tried meditation. I tried God, several of them. I tried 12-step programs. I tried soul retrievals and magic healing stones. I even tried getting up at 4:30 in the morning to shine a red light bulb on my tummy and listen to high-energy music for an hour (yes, it's weird and no, it didn't work). I finally had to come to a frightening realization: I was going to be fat no matter what I did. As I saw it, I had two options, one of which wasn't really an option. The first, non-option, was to kill myself. I had considered it at various stages in my life and I understand the pain of suicidal depression. I really do know how some people can see suicide as the best way to end the pain. A member of my extended family chose that option, and I saw what it did to my mother. I simply could not put her through that again. So my second, and only real option, was to just accept the fact that I was going to be fat, deal with it and try to be happy.

So that was it. I was apparently destined to be fat, so I just gave up the struggle. I started eating foods that I actually liked – things like pizza! I could have never remembered the last time I had actually *enjoyed* some pizza. I would have either denied myself of it, or I would have eaten it, felt guilty about it and later run ten miles to make up for it. But during that time, I ate pizza and actually enjoyed it. And I ate ice cream. I was amazed to discover that I didn't want to eat the whole carton, just a bowl was sufficient, and I somehow knew when to stop. And I didn't berate myself for eating the ice cream or work out for hours to make up for it later. I started to exercise in ways that felt good to me. I gave up the gym (who needs all those mirrors, anyway?) and started going for walks outside. And I didn't work out every day. And I didn't berate myself for not working out every day. I just accepted the fact that I was going to be fat and I was just trying to be happy.

And then an amazing thing happened. Somehow, somewhere, some way over the next few months, 45 pounds just vanished. I have no idea when or where they went. I was generally wearing big stretchy dresses and skirts at the time and had thrown out my scale, so I had no objective indication of my weight loss. When I looked in the mirror I still saw the same fat me, so that wasn't any help, either. I only discovered this tidbit of information because I had gone in for my annual exam and the nurse said my weight out loud to herself after I stepped off the scale. (I had shut my eyes so as to not see the horrid number.)

So there I was, flabbergasted. Maybe I wasn't destined to be fat? So off I was again on my next weight-loss effort. "If I could lose 45 pounds by eating pizza and ice cream," I reasoned, "think how much I could lose if I actually tried!" Without giving a thought to the horror that was my twenties, I once again started watching what I ate and started seriously working out. But nothing changed. I even went back to the food and exercise program that had helped me lose weight in grad school, but I actually started getting bigger. By this time I was seriously ready to lose it. Not only was my body out of control, so was my life. I was working three day jobs, performing in a play every night in a town 45 miles

The School of Hard Knocks

from home, and had just won my first leading role in a feature film, which was going to start shooting the following week. I didn't have time to *sleep,* let alone prepare "healthy" meals and work out. So for the next month I completely surrendered and did the best that I could do. That "best that I could do" included fast-food drive-thru meals three times a day for a month. Yes, I did the "Super Size Me" experiment, but somehow I managed to lose seven pounds.

Now I am not advocating a McDonald's diet. I am not advocating any type of diet in particular. What I am suggesting – through my own experience and the experiences my clients have shared with me – is that in the grand scheme of things, it is less important *what* you eat or how much, and *how* you exercise or how much, than how you *think and feel* about what you eat or how much, and how you exercise or how much, and that *the actions and thoughts and feelings and beliefs are congruent.* We only ever do anything to get what we want, and we only ever want anything because we think having it will make us feel better. And if the doing and the thinking and feeling don't jibe, neither will our results.

The only constant is change.

- Heraclitus

2

There are no "Once and for All – Forever and All Time" Solutions

I AM GOING TO GO OUT ON A LIMB HERE AND GUESS that this isn't the first weight-loss book you've picked up. Why is that? Don't you just need one? Don't you just need one book to tell you how much of what kind of foods to eat or what kind of exercises to do for your body? Don't you just need one psychologically based self-help book to tell you that you're eating because you are bored or lonely or angry rather than eating because you are hungry, or that you are carrying extra weight to "protect" you from your intimacy issues? Don't you just need one spiritually based self-help book to tell you all you need to do is say affirmations, think happy thoughts, meditate, turn it all over to God and He'll take care of the rest? The reason that the vast majority of weight-loss programs are ineffective – especially in the long term – is that they are incomplete. It's *ALL* true. Diet, exercise, psychology and spirituality are all important considerations. Yet these programs are not only incomplete, they leave out the most important, fundamental element: we do all this crap to get the body we think we want because we think getting it will make us happy.

So, before we go any further, I'd like to play a game of twenty questions. I encourage you to grab a notebook and actually work through these questions now. I, myself, have a tendency to just read through

There Are No "Forever and All Time" Solutions

books and answer the questions in my head. But I've learned the value of slowing down. By taking the time to really think about and write out the answers, you connect with yourself on a deeper level. And that's exactly who you need to connect with – YOU. YOU are the expert in the subject that is your own life. YOU are the one living in your body. YOU are the only one who knows how it feels to be you - physically, mentally, emotionally and spiritually. YOU are the common denominator in every weight-loss program you've ever tried, so grab a notebook. I'll wait.

Question #1: What do you want?
You want something. You wouldn't have picked up this book otherwise. What is it? Write it down. Be as specific as you can. Do not judge it.

Question #2: Why do you want it?
This is important. If what you want is "to lose weight," the desire and motivation to do so will feel

very different to you if you want to lose weight because your doctor says you have diabetes and "you should," than it will feel if you want to lose weight because you want to "look good" for your wedding.

Question #3: How will you know if you get it?

What is your indicator of success? Going back to the "lose weight" example, how will you know if and when you've met your goal? If you are working to lose weight because your doctor said so, how do you know when you've accomplished it? Are you simply looking at the number of pounds lost? Or are you looking to have other medical markers, such as blood pressure or cholesterol, fall within certain ranges? If you want to lose weight because you want to "look good" for your wedding, how will you know you've arrived? Is it a certain number on a scale or a dress size? Is it how you look to yourself in the mirror? Is it a reaction from your fiancé? What is it? There are many different indicators of success; just write down the first thing or things that come to mind.

There Are No "Forever and All Time" Solutions

Question #4: Is it reasonable or realistic to want what you want?

There is no judgment in this question. Furthermore, "reasonable" and "realistic" are subjective. It's not my place to tell you what's reasonable or realistic. It's just that if you're a five–foot, two-inch-tall woman and you want to grow to be a six-foot-tall supermodel, you're going to have more obstacles to overcome than if you want to run an eight-minute mile.

Question #5: Do you know how to get it?

Do you even know where to start? Do you have the information that might get you there?

Question #6: Have you had it before?

If so, how did it feel?

Question #7: Have you tried to get it before?

List everything you've tried. If you haven't tried getting it before, why haven't you? Is this simply a new want or has it not been important to you before? If it hasn't been important before, what changed to make it important to you?

Question #8: Have you succeeded in getting it before?
How did you feel about succeeding? Were you happy? Did *it* make you happy, specifically?

Question #9: What worked?
List what worked. If it worked, why did you stop? Did *it* quit working? Did *you* get bored, discouraged, too busy, or whatever and quit working it?

Question #10: Does it still work now?
If so, why aren't you doing it?

Question #11: Have you tried to get it before and failed?
How did you feel? What did you think?

There Are No "Forever and All Time" Solutions

Question #12: What didn't work?
List everything you've tried that didn't work. Why do you think it didn't work?

Question #13: Could it work now?
Are you in a different place physically, mentally, emotionally and/or spiritually that would be conducive to this method working?

Question #14: Do you <u>believe</u> you can get it?
This is probably one of the most important questions. If you've tried several approaches to getting whatever it is that you want and have failed, it's easy to get to the place where you just don't believe anymore that you can get it. Well, as Henry Ford said, "whether you think you can or you think you can't, either way you're right." So, if you don't believe you can get what you want, that's going to be the first thing you'll have to address.

Question #15: How do you feel about getting it?
Does it excite you? Does is depress you? What does the thought of getting it *feel* like?

Question #16: How do you feel about not having it yet?
Is it no big deal? Is it frustrating or demoralizing? What does the thought of not having it yet *feel* like?

Question #17: How determined are you to get it?
What are you willing to do to get it? What are you *not* willing to do?

Question #18: What is the worst thing that could happen if you don't get it?
Is it really the end of the world? It's okay if you say yes.

Question #19: What is the payoff for not having it?
What are you gaining by staying stuck where you are? Are there benefits to not getting it? For example, are your weight issues keeping you from dealing with

There Are No "Forever and All Time" Solutions

something else? Or are they giving you something in particular you don't believe you would otherwise have?

Question #20: What is stopping you?

So, how was that? If you were counting, you probably saw that I asked more than twenty questions. But did you learn anything interesting? If not, no biggie. I just wanted to get things stirred up inside of you so that you are clear about where you are in this whole process. I'm sure you noticed that several questions ask what you think or feel or believe about what you want. That's because our psychological, emotional and spiritual state really is just as important - if not slightly more so - than our physical state. And our physical state really is just as important - if not slightly more so - than our psychological, emotional and spiritual state. Yes, that's right – *it really is both ways.* The reason that it is both ways is because *YOU are both ways.* You are a physical being living in a physical world and you're going to have to deal with that. You are also a psychological, emotional and spiritual being and you're going to have to deal with that, too. Moreover, YOU are not a constant. You change with every breath you take. Every second, millions of cells in your body die and new ones are born. You change with every thought you think. You are changing by reading these words, and I am changing by writing them. You are constantly changing, just like that same damned river you can never step into twice. Sometimes you're a little more physical, and sometimes you're a little more psychological, emotional and spiritual. I like to think of it like a jazz band. Let the drums be exercise and the bass, food. Let the keyboards be your emotional and psychological state and the horns, your spirit. They all work together in perfect rhythm and harmony to play the song that is uniquely you. Your song reflects your state of being. But you know jazz players – they love their solos. So sometimes, for 32 measures, it really is just about the food. And at other

There Are No "Forever and All Time" Solutions

times, it might really be just about your perception of a troubling situation. But even when one instrument is taking center stage, the others are still quietly playing in the background for support. And ultimately, all the instruments always come back together to continue your song.

And that's the point. The song that is your state of being is the thing to focus on. And although the phrase "state of being" sounds all emotional and spiritual, your true, complete state of being is also very much physical. And focusing only on the physical is also incomplete. The trick is to look at (or listen to) the big picture and try to bring it all into harmony. When the way you *act* with food and exercise is congruent with what you *think* about food and exercise, is congruent with how you *feel* about food and exercise, is congruent with what you *believe* about food and exercise, and the whole experience is *making your state of being happy*, you will see results. If something is out of whack, you will ultimately be disappointed. The results won't come, they won't last, or you'll be miserable in the process. And if you're miserable in the process, you know you're on the wrong path because you started this whole thing to get something you wanted because you thought having it would . . . make you happy.

A bird does not sing because it has an answer.
It sings because it has a song.

~ Chinese Proverb

3

Happy Happy – Joy Joy

L̲ET'S TAKE A CLOSER LOOK AT THIS STATEMENT I KEEP repeating: *You only ever want anything because you think having it will make you happy.* I can hear the comments already. Someone somewhere is offering up some situation that seems to contradict this statement. But I challenge you to look deeply to see if, at the very bottom of it all, the motivation isn't to be happy. For instance, let's say you're in a job you hate. You still get up every day and go. Why? The paycheck. Why? To pay the rent. Why? So you have a roof over your head. Why? It's better than being homeless. Sometimes the choice seems to be the lesser of two evils, but you're always choosing the one you ultimately think will make you happier. Take a moment now to really ponder this statement. Again, the statement is: *You only ever want anything because you think having it will make you happy.* Think about different events and circumstances in your life and see if it isn't true. You're always doing the best you can with what you have in any given moment, and you're always doing the best you can to be happy. Now someone might argue that this theory doesn't hold up in the face of selfless acts. What is a selfless act, anyway? Don't you "do good" in the world because on some level you think that makes you a good person, and thinking of yourself as a good person makes you happy? And if there are such things as true selfless acts, isn't the act then coming from a place higher than yourself, a place of Divinity and Universal Good? And isn't that the ultimate expression of happiness anyway? Connection with *That*? This happiness thing is important because it is an indication of your state of being. And your state of being is the single most important factor in achieving any success, let alone weight loss.

Again, I ask, if weight loss is so simple, why is there an entire industry around it? If it's simply a matter of "calories in versus calories out," shouldn't we all have the bodies we desire? Nutritional information is the easiest thing in the world to find. Not only do we have Google, but now, thanks to new legislation, caloric and nutritional information is posted on drive-thru menus. The caloric expenditures of various physical activities are also easy to come by. We've got countless books and charts and, again, our friend Google. But you know by instinct and observation, if not by trial and error, that your body's shape and size isn't simply a "calories in versus calories out" equation. There's this mysterious thing called metabolism. Why else could all those skinny minis eat so freely and enjoy dessert while you suffer in silence with your salads? And now there are various "scientific" diets promising to help you "master" your metabolism. There are diets designed to help you identify your "type" and eat accordingly. There are diets based on using the glycemic index to balance your blood sugar. There are diets helping you with your hormones and diets helping you cleanse and detoxify your body. And don't forget the fitness programs. There are circuit training, interval training, and plyometric cardio fusion programs, all designed to increase your basal metabolic rate. Some "experts" promote eating *before* exercise, while others maintain that eating *after* you work out is most effective. The thing is, though, *no one* and I mean *no one* really understands metabolism and how it works. If anyone did, we'd all know it by now. It would be as simple as taking aspirin for a headache – problem solved. So I'll offer up my own theory on metabolism;

why not, right? Based on my own experience with my own body, and the experiences my clients have shared with me, I have come to believe that your "metabolism" is simply *the rate at which that wonderful energy of Life Force moves through you*. In other words, it's your *state of being*. When I am "aligned," – when my actions are congruent with my thoughts, are congruent with my feelings, are congruent with my beliefs, and I am happy – I seem to have a nuclear metabolism. *It truly does not matter* what I eat or how much, or what I choose to do for exercise or how much; my body looks more and more like the body I want. And when I'm out of alignment, *it truly does not matter* what I eat or how much, or what I choose to do for exercise or how much; my body moves further and further away from what I want. It's that simple. Now my only caveat to that is this: *only you know if you're in alignment or not.* I can't know, or do, it for you. No one can. It has to come from within. Only you know what you really think and feel and believe about food, exercise, yourself and life in general. Only you know if you're feeling connected to Yourself and your Source. Only you know if you're acting in a way that's congruent to your beliefs. Only you know if you're happy or not, and only you know what truly makes you happy.

So how do you "master" this metabolism called your state of being? You remember that you are a great jazz song, and you try to keep all the instruments in rhythm and harmony. Just keep in mind that those jazz players love their solos. You'll have times when the keyboards just want to lay it down. Don't freak out. Just try to make the best song out of it that you can. And remember that even when there is a solo going on, the other instruments are still playing, even if they are playing quietly, for support.

In case you're getting tired of the music analogy, let's get back to you. There's the physical you – the food, the exercise, the how you physically feel in your body – and there's the non-physical you – your thoughts, feelings, emotions and spirit. When everything's all lined up, life is good. You're in the zone. Life Force can flow through you freely and effectively. Let's now take a moment to discuss each of these aspects we're trying to align.

If you are going to worry, don't do it.
If you do it, don't worry.

~ Don Ward

4

Let's Get Physical

Food. Big subject, filled with lots of thoughts, feelings, emotions and complications. Wait a minute. We were supposed to be discussing the physical body. That's right. Okay, food, but food as it relates to aligning you to Yourself and being happy. The answers to your big food questions are already within you. Are you the type of person who likes "food plans"? Do you like having someone else tell you when, what and how much to eat? If you like the structure and routine and not having to think about it, or if it makes you feel safe, then by all means, pick your food plan and stick with it. If food plans (or diets) make you crazy, then forget them. Eat intelligently, do the best you can, let yourself off the hook and get on with it. If you have special dietary needs due to allergies or doctor's orders, try to find a way to focus on what you *can* eat, rather than on what you *can't,* and really enjoy what you can eat. Three square meals a day? Several mini-meals spread out over the day? Only you can be the judge of that. Does one way help you feel better physically over the other? Does one way help you feel better mentally and emotionally over the other? *The best way to think about food is to remember its original intention – to nourish your body.* Listen to your body; it will tell you what it wants and needs. If it really wants a cookie, you can give your body a cookie

Let's Get Physical

without being fearful of it. When you surrender to the idea that your body is your friend rather than something to be feared and hated, you'll be amazed to discover that sometimes your body really does want a salad and you'll be happy to feed it that, too. You will discover that you actually enjoy the salad rather than resent it. Later on I'll be sharing some tips and tools that have helped me with the whole food thing, but right now let's move on to exercise.

Okay, exercise. Be like Nike and just do it. That may sound harsh, but if you listen to your body, you will discover that it really *wants* to move. My attitude on exercise comes not from my lifetime of constant body obsession, but from my eight years as a Certified Classical Pilates instructor. Over the years I've had countless clients walk into my studio, many of whom were in their fifties, sixties and seventies. One day, one of my clients brought her 94-year-old mother-in-law to see me, and it was heartbreaking. She could barely move. She had lost almost all of her strength and flexibility. Now I know what you're thinking:

"Give the woman a break – she's 94, for crying out loud." But her condition isn't a necessary result of aging. It's a necessary result of inactivity. So if you want to be able to walk, stand up and sit down by yourself, feel good in your body and have any kind of quality of life in your later years – move your body! You don't have to become a triathlete or a master yogi. Just start and keep moving. If you've been inactive for a while or if you are heavy, it may very well be uncomfortable at first – trust me, I really do know. But find something that you can tolerate – it's even better if you can enjoy it – and just do it. Start small. Do one small thing every day. Overcoming inertia is the hardest thing. Once you've done that, it gets easier. Remember, we aren't exercising to lose weight. We are moving to get our physical bodies into alignment with the Life Force that moves through us. It's like cleaning the sludge out of your engine. I had a friend whose job was to tune up Porsches. Do you know how you tune up a Porsche? You take it out on the open highway and really open it up. Again, don't

Let's Get Physical

panic. I am not suggesting you go full force. Just wiggle your toes, move your joints and get your blood flowing through your veins. Your body will respond. Your body will thank you. Moving your body will start to feel good. Then you will start moving your body *because* it feels good. And remember what this whole thing is about? *Feeling good!* Feeling good physically, as well as mentally, emotionally and spiritually.

Now if you're someone who exercises compulsively, that's something to look at, too. The premise of this book is that happy calories don't count, but neither does unhappy exercise. And only you know how you really feel about exercise. One woman's discipline is another woman's compulsion. It's not the exercise that counts, but rather the motivation and feelings behind it and whether or not that activity brings you into alignment with your highest self. If you continue to run on a treadmill every morning even though it makes you feel like a caged hamster in a wheel, you aren't doing yourself any favors. Not only will your body start to give you signs of its displeasure, such as stress fractures or pulled ligaments, you will eventually discover diminishing returns from your efforts. (See, I *knew* that econ degree would be useful someday.) The most effective way to get the body you think you want is to *enjoy it*. Enjoy what you feed it and enjoy how you move it. Rest it when it needs it. If you are trying to achieve a very specific look or goal, by all means do your research and eat and exercise in a way you think will help you achieve that. Just know that when you are dialed in and everything is aligned, anything you choose to eat and anything you to choose to do for exercise is effective. When you are out of alignment and there's static in the signal, no diet or exercise program is ultimately effective.

Now here's an interesting point that many psychologically and spiritually based weight-loss books fail to mention, or if they do mention it at all, it's barely a footnote. Sometimes the fastest way to get into better psychological, emotional and spiritual tune is through changing your diet and/or exercising! Greatly simplified, the fundamental premise of most psychological and spiritual weight-loss programs is that by changing your habitual patterns of thought, you can effect more lasting changes in your behavior and your body. But sometimes you're crabby simply because you're hungry! *It goes both ways.* Yes, your thoughts, feelings and perceptions create a state of mind through which you see the world. And if you change your thoughts, feelings and perceptions, you see the world differently. And hopefully from this new vantage point, you discover inner peace. Behaviors may or may not change. As the Zen saying goes, "Before enlightenment, chop wood and carry water. After enlightenment, chop wood and carry water." You might still get up and get on that treadmill every morning. But this new perspective helps you *feel better.* Remember, that's the whole point of everything. This time, on the treadmill, you no longer feel like a caged hamster in a wheel. You are disciplined rather than compulsed. But *feeling better* isn't always achieved through your mind alone! Feeling better is also affected by your physical body. Sometimes it's hard to think happy thoughts and see the beauty of the world if you've got a raging headache. And that headache could simply be the result of too much coffee and not enough water. Sometimes an afternoon headache is the result of a blood-sugar crash. Sometimes that afternoon headache is a result of sitting at a computer too long, causing diminished blood flow to your brain. So get up and go for a walk. Get fresh air and clear your head. Clearing your head can be just as much a physical process as it is a psychological, emotional and spiritual process. And if you've got a clear head physically, it's much easier to do the psychological, emotional and spiritual work you might also need to do.

That they may have a little peace,
even the best dogs
are compelled to snarl occasionally.

- William Feather

5

Let's Get Meta-Physical

Psychology, emotions and spirituality. I'm sure that someone out there would be happy to define them as three distinct aspects of self. But to me, practically speaking, they're all the same thing. Each is so intimately tied to the others, it's impractical and futile to try to tease them apart to specify which aspect you might need to address at any given time. I just lump them all together as the touchy-feely, non-physical and sometimes "airy-fairy" stuff. As I mentioned before, the fundamental premise of the non-physical is that your perception creates your reality. Nowhere is this more clearly and easily illustrated than with the optical illusion. Take a piece of paper and draw a square. Go ahead, get out a piece of paper and draw a square. I'll wait. Now draw a second square a little higher and a little farther over to the right than the first square, but make sure the squares overlap. Now draw lines connecting the corners of the squares to make a cube. Now stare at it. Keep staring at it. What happens? *It changes!* Sometimes it looks like the cube is reaching up and to the right and sometimes, when you shift your gaze, it looks like the cube is coming forward down and to the left. But the cube isn't really going anywhere at all – it's just a piece of paper with a bunch of lines on it! There, I've just distilled years of therapy and everything ever written about psychology and spirituality into a single analogy. You're welcome. So what does all this mean? It means that we're the only ones who ascribe any meaning to anything. Nothing is a problem unless you choose to perceive it as a problem. And since you're the perceiver, you can change what you focus on. And by changing what you focus on, you change your experience. The problematic cube may not change at all. It's still the same piece of paper with the same bunch of lines on it. But *your experience of it* can change. And all of this non-physical stuff is about changing your experience for the better. Remember, the whole point of all of this is to be happy. We want what we want because we think getting it will make us happy.

So if you are already working with the physical components of weight loss and you aren't seeing the results that you want, something else in your alignment is mucked up. You've got to align everything – your actions, your thoughts, your feelings and beliefs – to get into that sublime state of being where it all comes together easily and effectively. If you are taking action with a diet-and-exercise program and things are slow to move, it's time to deal with the non-physical.

So here we go. Make a list of all the things you're upset about and get over it. Forgive your mother. Forgive your lovers. Forgive your father. Forgive your children. Forgive anyone and everyone who's ever done you wrong. Forgive yourself. Get professional help if you need it. Get spiritual help if you need it. Claim your power. Surrender control. Spend five minutes alone every day in peace and quiet. Make lists of the good things in your life. See the glass as half full. Write down 25 things you like about yourself. I know it's hard, but do it. Make sure a couple of those things you like about yourself are physical. I know - that's hard, too. But do you know what I discovered? I have a *great* head of hair! It's a deep chestnut brown and long and healthy. I also have big brown eyes! And thanks to my dad, I've got this great olive skin that doesn't burn in the sunshine! Quit looking in the mirror! Or if you must, focus on the things you like, ignore the things you don't. Mirrors don't reflect physical reality, anyway – they reflect your state of mind. To improve your state of mind, Louise Hay promotes a practice she calls "mirror work." You're supposed to look at yourself in the mirror and say to yourself, "I love you. I really love you." And she encourages you to use your name, too. I think that's great. I really do. But sometimes that's impossible. So I think that when necessary, it's just as good, if not better, to *not* look in the mirror and to *not* hate yourself. Quit hating yourself! Notice every time you have a negative thought about yourself. Think of what a best friend would say to that negative thought. Or simply reject the thought. Even better, *transform* the thought. Say affirmations. Get a mantra. Breathe. Spend time "being" in nature. Make a *decision* to be happy. You only have this one life. *Decide* that you're going to enjoy it! Quit looking at magazines - all the pictures are Photoshopped, anyway. Quit reading tabloid headlines – they're just more negative energy. Whose idea was it, anyway, to create the most unflattering pictures possible of celebrities and flaunt them in supermarket checkout lines? It's mean, and looking at those pictures doesn't contribute to *your* state of being in a positive way, either. Even Michelangelo's *David* is imperfect from just the right angle. The *David* was originally intended to be placed upon the buttress of the cathedral in Florence, forty feet above anyone looking at him. Consequently, Michelangelo sculpted his proportions with this in mind. So now, when you are looking at him in the Galleria dell'Accademia museum, his hand is too big and his eyes are too deeply set. Quit sizing up other people, and you will quit sizing up yourself. Quit judging other people, and you will quit judging yourself. Let people live in peace. Start appreciating other people, and you will start to appreciate yourself. Practice random acts of kindness. Tell someone you love something specific that you appreciate about them. Compliment someone in the grocery store – tell them you like their hair or their outfit or whatever.

Let's Get Meta-Physical

When you bless the beauty you see in others (rather than resent it), you will begin to see the beauty in yourself. Remember that other people's actions and words say more about them than they do about you. Remember that everyone is just doing the best they can with what they have available to them in any given moment. Pet your cat. Be the person your dog thinks you are. Read uplifting books. Listen to music. Sometimes there's no better way to move energy than to bang your head to eighties rock. Is that enough? For now, anyway? Like I said, there are entire books devoted to how to deal with the touchy-feely, non-physical and sometimes "airy-fairy" stuff. The point of them all being, how to release the pain and resistance in your life and to just be happy – authentically happy. For this book, I'll simply elaborate on some of the tools that have helped me deal with both the physical and the non-physical.

The holiest of all spots on earth is where an ancient hatred has become a present love.

~ A Course in Miracles

6

Tools of the Trade

THE MOST PROFOUND THING THAT HAS HELPED ME deal with my physical body is the work of Joseph Pilates. I tread lightly as I mention this because now the term "Pilates" really doesn't mean anything. The industry has been deregulated for a decade and thanks to celebrity devotees, "Pilates" has become synonymous with marketing dollars. If you see the word "Pilates", chances are very high that at best it is a diluted form of, or at worst it has nothing to do with, the method that changed my life. And when I say that Pilates changed my life, I don't mean that the exercise program helped me lose weight and change my body. It did do that, but the most profound and unexpected thing that Pilates did for me was to *connect me to my body.*

When you abuse your body, through starvation, overeating, over exercising, lack of movement or in any other way, you disconnect from it. That's how you handle the pain and keep going. In this day and age and in this country, if you are connected to your body you cannot starve it. It won't let you and you won't want to. If you are connected to your body, you are not seduced by a cookie if you don't really want it. If you are connected to your body, you simply cannot keep eating until there is literally no more room in your stretched-out stomach. If you are connected to your body, you won't run eight miles with blood

Tools of the Trade

blisters on your feet. The body sends you pain signals to stop, and since you're connected to it and listening, you stop. If you are connected to your body, you will feel it ask to wiggle and stretch and you'll answer. Remember when I said that the key to that magical state of being (and metabolism) is to align your physical, psychological, emotional and spiritual aspects? Well, Pilates helped me align myself to my body and that is a *huge* deal.

My little Hello Kitty notebooks are the other main tool that I use to deal with my physical body. I use them to deal with my food, but I use them in a psychological way, so I think they make a good transition subject. Hello Kitty. I know I'm a grown woman, but I love her. There's something about the proportions of her face and her little expression that makes me happy. (Remember, that's the whole point of everything – Happy! Happy! Happy!) So I allow myself some whimsy and I buy small, three-by-five-inch, 35-sheet Hello Kitty notebooks. I start a new one each month, a page for each day. And on that page I write down anything and everything I eat or drink all day long. I write the time, what I ate and about how much. I know, some of you are probably thinking that's a bit crazy and/or compulsive, but it really does work! I eat something, I write it down and I never have to think about it again! And I don't *not* eat something just because I'd have to write it down. My rule is that I can eat anything I want as long as I write it down. It's amazing! For years I'd mentally and emotionally hang on to everything I ever ate, logging calories and fat grams, trying to balance it all out with my exercise. Now I can just write it down and forget it. It's still written down in the notebook; I haven't "lost" it. I can still go back and look over everything I've ever eaten for the past week or month or year if I so desire. But I never have. They just pile up in my desk drawer.

Another way little Miss Hello Kitty is such a great friend is that she is an early warning for me when something is out of whack (read *alignment*). I write down everything. And it's not when what I eat

Tools of the Trade

or how much I eat starts to change that's the problem. It's when what I start to *feel about* what or how much I eat starts to change, when I start *judging* what I write down in my little Hello Kitty notebook, that I know I've got something out of alignment going on. Then I just have to figure out what it is and deal with it.

Now I've never had this problem myself, but some people are simply unconscious of what and how much they eat. So if you think you fall into that category, a little food journal is wonderful help. You can't change the things you're unaware of, and a food journal is a great tool to raise your consciousness about your dietary habits. You can then see things objectively and notice if there's anything you'd like to change.

Speaking of dietary habits, let's discuss calories. Wikipedia defines a calorie as "a pre-SI metric unit of *energy*." Calories were first defined in 1824. A guy by the name of Nicolas Clément defined them as units of *heat.* I think that's fascinating. Calories aren't food, they are *energy* and *heat.* Conventional wisdom suggests that if you consume more calories than your body uses, your body will store that *energy and heat* as fat. Conventional wisdom also suggests that you use up *energy and heat* when you engage in physical activity such as exercise. Hmmm. Interesting. In what other activities might we engage that use *energy and heat*? What about crying, screaming and beating pillows? Have you ever heard the term *emotional energy*? What about *white-hot rage*? That's why I told you to make a list of everything you're upset about and get over it. That's why I told you to forgive anyone and everyone who's ever done you wrong. Holding on to anger and resentment is deadly. I have no scientific proof that repressed anger and resentment translate into fat (would you really want to risk it?), but I do know that *holding on to anger and resentment will keep you out of alignment* and that *will* keep you from getting what you want. So do what you need to do – therapy, cry fests, scream at the top

Tools of the Trade

of your lungs in your car, headbang to Iron Maiden, whatever – just move the energy and *let it go*!

I have a client who can't let it go. She insists she's in the right. She can argue her point every which way to Sunday, and she *is* in the right. But is being *right* more important than being *happy*? What's the point of being right if it's making you miserable (and out of alignment and fat)? Letting it go isn't a statement of weakness. It's empowering. *You* are the source of power in your own life. Forgiveness isn't something you do for another person, it's a gift you give to yourself. Mark Twain wrote, "Forgiveness is the fragrance the violet sheds on the heel that has crushed it." And that fragrance is the sweet smell of your personal alignment.

Letting it go isn't only about giving up repressed anger and resentment. I have a friend who would definitely fall into the heavy category. Last time we met for coffee I made an interesting observation. We hugged, I asked her how she was, and she immediately launched into all this drama. And it's not so much that she's a drama queen, she's not. It's that everything is so *heavy*. She ascribes so much *meaning* to *everything* and everything is *such a big deal*, and she has all these expectations of the way things should be that aren't. You know how they talk about "energy vampires," people who seem to feed on and suck up all your energy? Well, she was an "energy oppressor." It was suffocating and I wanted to tell her to lighten the hell up! But I didn't. I kept my mouth shut. Later it occurred to me that if she lightened up in her attitudes about life, she would probably lighten up in her body as well.

So how do you lighten up? You surrender control. You can only control two things anyway: your thoughts and your actions. But in controlling your thoughts and your actions, you have great power. I like to ask the question, "What *can* I do?" It's easy to ask, "What can I do?" with the emphasis being on the *I* or the *do*. The questions, "What can *I* do?" and "What can I *do*?" are disempowering. They come from a mentality of powerlessness and

Tools of the Trade

victimization. I like to focus on the *can*. I *can* drink more water today. I *can* go for a walk. I *can* stop and take a deep breath. I *can* choose to ignore that comment. I *can* choose to look at this situation in another way. I *can* choose to keep looking for a way to look at this situation that will bring me peace. I *can* choose to give this other person the benefit of the doubt. I *can* choose to make amends. I *can* choose to focus on the positive. And when you really *can't* do anything at all, and you really *can't* think any thought that will make you feel better – be *willing*. Willingness is the greatest gift you can give yourself. I *am willing* to be wrong (just this once). I *am willing* to let go of the pain. I *am willing* to love myself. I *am willing to be willing* to not hate myself. Willingness puts you into a state of non-resistance, a place of surrender where the Universe can step in to help you out. And when the Universe steps in, miracles happen.

You are what you think -
Not what you think you are.

– Bruce MacLelland

7

Repeat After Me: "All Is Well in My World"

STATEMENTS SUCH AS "I *CAN* CHOOSE TO FOCUS ON the positive" and "I *am willing* to let go of the pain" are affirmations. Affirmations aren't weird or scary or "airy-fairy," they're simply statements you make to yourself. And you're making statements to yourself all the time. Every time you look in the mirror and see yourself as less than, you are saying an affirmation to yourself, even if it isn't verbalized. Every time you judge what or how much you eat, you are saying an affirmation to yourself. Every time you say to yourself, "I just don't have the time to exercise," you are making an affirmation. You affirm all the time, whether you're aware of it or not. The trick is to become aware and make these affirmations work in your favor! How do you do that?

There are two fundamental aspects of affirmations upon which you need to focus to make them effective tools for positive change. First, you need to phrase your statements in a positive way, and second, the statements need to make you feel better. It's easy to focus on the weight you want to lose. And focusing on the weight you want to lose is helping it stay there! If you are looking in the mirror and repeating to yourself over and over that you no longer have cellulite on your thighs, what are you really focusing on? The cellulite. And by focusing on it, it keeps hanging around. Focus on what you want, not on what you don't want. So focus on lean, shapely, toned legs. Forget the fat and quit looking in the mirror! Or if you must, look at the lines of muscle definition that are forming and focus on that.

Not only is it necessary for you to phrase your affirmative statements in ways that focus on what you're trying to achieve (you aren't trying to lose weight, you are trying to be fit, healthy, strong, flexible and in alignment with Yourself), it's necessary that these statements make you *feel better*. Remember? That's the whole point of everything! The power of affirmations lies not in their words. It's not like "Open, Sesame," magic words delivering magical results. *The power of affirmations lies in the way the words make you feel.*

Let's say you are well over 200 pounds and you want to change your thoughts and your self-talk to help you change your body. Let's say you choose the statement "I am a beautiful size six" as an affirmation. I am not suggesting that a six is any type of ideal size, I simply like the alliteration. If you just repeat this statement over and over by rote, it does nothing for you. The words "I am a beautiful size six" are not magical. The words themselves will not do a darned thing. Moreover, the words "I am a beautiful size six" have the potential to make you feel even *worse.* If you cannot imagine that you are a size six (let alone beautiful) to begin with, saying it over and over just creates contradictory energy. You can't believe that it's true because it's too far of a reach. You can't see how that significant of a change in your body could come without significantly - and painfully - changing your dietary and/or exercise habits. You can't emotionally see yourself as a size six, so energetically the whole thing backfires. You've got static in the signal, things are mucked up – you are out of alignment with Yourself.

If, on the other hand, you *can* imagine that you are a size six and the phrase, "I am a beautiful size six" *excites and energizes* you, then it's worth using as an affirmation. It's the excitement and energizing (or peace-giving) aspect of the statement, not the words

Repeat After Me, "All is well in my world."

themselves, that is the magic. By being excited and energized and at peace and *feeling better,* you align your energy emotionally and spiritually. And do you know the best thing about emotional and spiritual alignment? It *inspires* you to physical action! Suddenly you will "feel like" eating more vegetables. You will "feel like" doing yoga or going for a swim. All the physical changes you might need to make to become a size six are effortless and painless.

So what do you do if you're well over 200 pounds and you *can't* imagine that you're a size six? You don't use that affirmation. You find a different one that works. You find a statement you can believe. You discover a phrase, stated in such a way that it focuses on what you want, that does make you feel better, if not excited and energized. For me personally, my affirmations need to stay general. The minute I start getting too focused on details, I get mucked up. By creating an affirmation focusing on specific details of my body that I'd like to change, I am by definition stating that my body is not perfect the way it already is. And when I get into that frame of mind, I'm instantly out of alignment with myself. So for me, I need to say things like, "every day my body becomes closer and closer to the vision I hold of it."

Now some would argue that the statement "every day my body becomes closer and closer to the vision I hold of it" means that I will never get the body I think I want. There are people who will say that for affirmations to be effective, you need to state what you want as if you already have it in the present. These people will say that if you say an affirmation like "I am going to weigh 150 pounds" you will never achieve your goal. They say that this is because "the Universe takes us at our word." They say that if you keep repeating to yourself "I am going to weigh 150 pounds," the Universe then says, "Okay, you are *going to.*" You are *going to*, you never actually do. Well, I say that the Universe takes us at our *feeling*. The words are not the magic. It's the alignment that the words have the potential to bring you that's the magic. Oftentimes the best affirmation is to simply breathe. Take a deep breath and stop that habitual negative thought you were about to think. You'll instantly feel better and, again, that's the ultimate point anyway. My personal favorite affirmation is, "There's enough." There's enough time. There's enough money. There's enough love. There's enough. I'm enough.

Another of my favorite affirmations is Jeff Goldblum's famous line in *Jurassic Park*, "Life finds a way." I'm old enough to remember when Mount St. Helens blew her top. And being from the state of Washington, it was a really big deal. Pictures of the eruption and its destruction were everywhere. Images of trees knocked over by mudslides, the mountain with half its face missing, and cars covered with ash were the staple of the evening news for months. I even had to do a report on it for school. But now, years later, the deer are back. Flowers grow. Snow caps the mountain in the wintertime. The forests have returned. Nature is always right. *Life finds a way.* Even grass, given the slightest opportunity, will grow through concrete. Like Marianne Williamson says, "There has never been a storm that has not passed." The sun really does come up every morning. It may be cloudy (especially in the Pacific Northwest), but the sun really is there. Those are some of the thoughts that have helped me through my darkest nights.

So how do you know if you're succeeding? What is your indicator of success? Is it a number on a scale? We know that scales don't accurately reflect your true state of health or beauty. You can line up three women, all the same height and weight, and they can look completely different. Is it a dress size? By now I'm sure you've discovered that women's sizing is anything but standard. One designer's size twelve is another designer's size eight. Is it what you see in the mirror? We know that mirrors do not reflect physical reality; what they reflect changes depending on your mood. Is it a tape measure? That's probably the most objective, but it's also just another number about which you can obsess. To me, the most important indicator of success is *how you feel.* Remember that we only want the bodies we think we want because we think that having them will make us happy. If what you are doing isn't making you happy, either you won't see results or they will be short-lived. When you can find that magical place of alignment in which your actions are congruent with your thoughts, are congruent with your feelings, are congruent with your beliefs, and everything is making you happy, you enter a zone and your body responds. It transforms easily and effortlessly into the body you've always wanted. And when any piece of the puzzle is out of place, your body can't get to be, or stay, the way you want it to be. Alignment is all about your connection with Yourself and your Source – physically, mentally, emotionally and spiritually. So rather than focus on outside indicators to measure the success you may or may not be achieving in your weight-loss efforts, let your body itself be an indicator of your alignment. That's the greatest gift it can give you.

Just when the caterpillar thought life was over,
it became a butterfly.

- Unknown

8

The Fifth Element

I LIKE THE ANALOGY OF THE JAZZ BAND BECAUSE IT reminds me not to panic. If one instrument, or aspect of self, suddenly wants to solo – it's okay. If I'm trying to figure things out and deal with them, but I'm still freaking out a bit about my food – it's okay. That bass player can have his darned solo. The instruments will eventually come back together to continue the song. Sometimes it's the fighting against what's going on with you that makes - and keeps - the song out of rhythm or tune. Sometimes it's better to just let the guy solo and get it out of his system. The other instruments haven't stopped playing. They are still there for support, and they will ultimately pull him back into the groove with the rest of them.

Another analogy I find helpful is that of The Fifth Element. Understand that you are a conduit of Universal Life Force and the rate at which this force flows through you is your metabolism. But the conduit that is You isn't a single, smooth, pipe-like concept. The conduit that is You is created from five elements - the physical elements of food and exercise, and the non-physical elements of thoughts, feelings, and beliefs. Imagine that these elements are rings, stacked one on top of the other. Order does not matter in this analogy. The energetic Life Force of your metabolism flows from your Universal Source through the five elements of You. When the elements

The Fifth Element

are perfectly aligned, energy can flow freely and powerfully. Just imagine the ending of the movie *The Fifth Element*, when all the power of Universal Good flows through the heroine as a powerful beam of Light to overcome the Darkness. If one or more of the elements is slightly off center, energy can't flow as freely or effectively. Our goal is to do the best we can, moment by moment, to keep that conduit open. If one of the elements can't lock into place because it is crusted over with repressed anger and resentment, we need to clean it up and let the anger and resentment go. If an element is out of place because of poor nutrition, or because of habitual negative self-talk, we need to address it so we can get that element back into alignment. We only struggle when we're misaligned. If you're struggling, do the best you can to identify which element is out of place, and do the work you need to do to get it back in line with the others. And yet, paradoxically, sometimes the key to getting that fifth element into alignment is to simply surrender the struggle. When the five elements are aligned, we've got the power of the Universe running through us freely and powerfully. And with that, anything is possible.

Never confuse motion for action.

– Hemingway

9

The Body Shop

THE GREATEST GIFT THE WORK OF JOSEPH PILATES HAS given me has been to connect me to my body. The greatest gift teaching Pilates has given me is the understanding that *no one* – I repeat, *no one* – has a "perfect" body. Most of my clients are just regular people who have heard that Pilates can help them deal with their back issues or what have you. Some of them are trying to lose weight, but most of them just want to stay active with an exercise method and a teacher that can help them deal with their specific goals, needs and/or limitations. Every now and again, I'll have a panicked moment of "less-than-ness" when a cute little size two missy in designer workout clothes walks through the door. But within five minutes, that feeling is gone. She may indeed look good, but I quickly discover that even she does not have a "perfect" body. She may have no strength or perhaps little flexibility or coordination. Or she might have scoliosis that is only noticeable upon close examination.

No one has a *perfect* body. Beauty may be in the eye of the beholder, but biomechanics are not. The best you can hope for is the perfect body for *you.* And the perfect body for *you* is based not only on things that are in your control, like your thoughts and your actions, but also on things over which you have no control, like your skeletal structure. You can intuitively surmise that not all bones are the same given the fact that people are different heights. But do you really know how individual bones are? I know this will be hard to grasp through words alone – it's much better if you can see it. But I'll try anyway. Think of a femur bone. That's your thigh bone, and it has a little bobble, called the trochanter, that angles off the top of it. The trochanter is the "ball" of the ball-and-socket joint that is your hip. And the size, shape, length and angle of that silly little bobble have *huge* implications for the range of motion in your hip joints, which affects the shape of your butt!

Because of the shape of my trochanters and how they fit into my pelvis, I can't sit criss-cross very well. (Indian-style is no longer politically correct, so those of you with young children will know "criss-cross applesauce.") It has nothing to do with the flexibility in my muscles. It has to do with my bones. And because of the way my bones are put together, I can sit like an "M" with my knees rolled in, feet kicked out to the side, and lay all the way back on the ground – something that horrifies most people. I have never been able to do the splits – I have always been about three inches off the ground. Again, it has nothing to do with my flexibility, it's the way my joints are built. So your range of motion is defined not only by the flexibility of your muscles, but also by your bone structure.

Why is your range of motion important to consider? Your range of motion helps define which muscles you engage and to what extent you engage them. Your muscles hold your bones together and if your bones are limiting your range of motion, they will limit the extent to which your muscles can engage (or stretch). Muscular engagement is important because that's what creates the nice, shapely tone of the muscles of your body. It sounds fairly obvious - you need to engage your muscles to tone them. But you'd be amazed at how easy it is to "cheat" and not work the muscles you think you're working. Most of the people I see doing that double straight leg lift to work the abdominals aren't really

The Body Shop

working their abdominal muscles at all! They do most of the work from their superficial hip-flexor muscles, which are the "hinge" muscles between the pelvis and the front of the leg. Consequently, those over-developed muscles begin to pull on the pelvis and the abdominal muscles remain weak. This often results in back pain and that lower tummy "pooch". Do you do endless hours of cardio and lift weights but still have "back fat"? Then it's a good bet that you're using your neck and traps to lift most of the weight. Are your triceps flabby despite hours of work? The slightest rotation of your humerus (your upper arm bone) affects how those muscles work, and how that bone is able to rotate is partly determined by how your shoulder joint is built. The same is true for the legs. A ballerina's "turnout" is developed through hard work, but her ability to develop the turnout is offered up in her bone structure. Some people just can't do dance plies or plie squats because their hip joints won't let them. And if they can't get their bones into those positions, they can't get certain specific muscle groups to work and tone up using those exercises.

So what do you do? You know that to tone a muscle you actually need to engage it. You watch your alignment (gee, there's that word again) and you try to feel the muscle that you're trying to tone up truly work. And if you find that doing certain exercises isn't letting you feel that specific muscle work because of structural limitations, try to find a different way to engage that muscle. Work with an objective observer if you can, a trainer or a physical therapist or a workout buddy. Sometimes the weak link in the chain is simply our own proprioception and we need an outside eye to help us. And if you're really adventurous, you'll try something like Structural Integration (Rolfing, Hellerwork, Myofascial Release).

Structural Integration focuses on working the connective tissues in the body to effect change in alignment, and I've seen amazing results. Sometimes, certain muscles can't engage because the bones can't

The Body Shop

get into a certain position. And those bones can't get into a certain position because other connective tissues are binding them up in their current alignment patterns. If the connective tissues binding up the alignment of the bones can be "unstuck," then the alignment of the bones, and consequently the engagement and tone of certain muscle groups, can change. I was amazed to discover that the insanely high arches in my feet were partially a result of some bound-up connective tissue. Once that was released, my feet, ankles, knees and hips started to work in better alignment (that magic word) and therefore, look better. I was also thrilled to discover that little dimples on your legs aren't always cellulite. Those, too, are sometimes signs of bound-up connective tissue.

I can get Rolfed and unbind stuck connective tissue until the cows come home, but I still can't change the shape of my femur bones. I guess that's the next miracle for me to try to manifest. If I succeed, I'll let you know. In the meantime, let us all remember to appreciate our bodies as the wonderful indicators of our physical, mental, emotional and spiritual alignment that they are. We only struggle when we're misaligned. When we're in that magical zone where we're connected, to ourselves and to our Source, our bodies easily and painlessly become more and more like the visions we hold in our heads. And we only want the bodies we think we want because we think having them will make us happy. So let's help our bodies out - be well and be happy.

If you meet someone who needs a miracle,
give them one of yours.

- Mary Augustine

10

In Other Words

Here are just a few more treasures that I've discovered along the way. Some I saw on greeting cards, some came along at just the right moment in an e-mail. And some of them are a mystery. I don't remember when or where I first heard them, but they've stuck with me somehow. I offer them up in hopes that they may bring you peace and encouragement as well.

Never place a period where God has placed a comma.
　～ Gracie Allen

No one really knows enough to be a pessimist.
　～ Norman Cousins

Blessed are those who have faith who cannot see.
　～ Jesus

At each stage of learning we must give up something, even if it is a way of life that we have always known.
　～ Ginevee, Australian Aborigine

Fall down seven times, get up eight.
　～ Buddhist Proverb

In Other Words

God Himself shall wipe away all tears.
~ A Course in Miracles

It is impossible to begin to learn that which one thinks one already knows.
~ Heraclitus

You are loved. If so, what else matters?
~ Edna St. Vincent Millay

When a rose and an orchid are side by side, is one more beautiful than the other?
~ Unknown

If you really want to be happy, nobody can stop you.
~ Sister Mary Tricky

You can learn more by climbing the same mountain one hundred times than by climbing one hundred different mountains.
~ Unknown

Happy Calories Don't Count

There will come a time when you believe everything is finished. That will be the beginning.
> ~ Louis L'Amour

Some of life's greatest lessons cannot be pried from books – they must be experienced in your bones.
> ~ Kobi Yamada

"What is the heaviest burden?" asked the child. "To have nothing to carry," answered the old man.
> ~ Unknown

Good Friend, always be open to the miracle of the second chance.
> ~ The Reverend David Stier

Give thanks for unknown blessings already on their way.
> ~ Native American Saying

In Other Words

To be a star you must shine your own light, follow your own path and do not worry about the darkness, for that is when stars shine the brightest.

~ Unknown

Fear knocked at the door. Faith answered. No one was there.

~ Inscription at Hind's Head Inn, England

May today there be peace within. May you trust your highest power that you are exactly where you are meant to be. May you not forget the infinite possibilities that are born of faith. May you use those gifts that you have received and pass on the love that has been given to you. May you be content knowing that you are a child of God. Let this presence settle into your bones and allow your soul the freedom to sing, dance, and to bask in the sun.

~ St. (Mother) Teresa

Happy Calories Don't Count

Look forward with faith. See only good in your future. Know that all things work together for your highest good. Know that God is taking care of everything, and watch with attentive interest as your highest and best unfolds. This will leave room for those wonderful surprises and unexpected events that make your life a joyous and educational adventure.

~ Marianne Williamson
quoting *Unity Magazine*

So that's it. That's what I've learned. With everything we go through to get our bodies the way we want them, we're really just doing it so we can be happy. How wonderful it was to discover that *happy* calories *don't* count, and *happy* exercise *does.* Remember that *unhappy* calories *do* count, and *unhappy* exercise *doesn't.* Be patient with yourself. Alignment is a moment-by-moment experience. Trust Yourself. Be well, and be happy.

Harnessing Alignment Produces a Powerful You™

Exercise your options!

I hope you enjoyed this book. For free videos and other resources please visit:

>   www.happycaloriesdontcount.com.

Food for thought!

Let me know how I can help you. Please send your questions, triumphs and hurdles to:

>   askcarmela@happycaloriesdontcount.com.

In the meantime…

Be well and be happy!

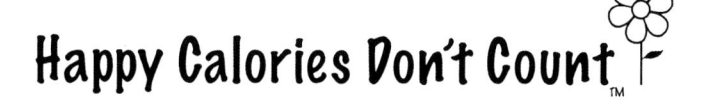

Happy Calories Don't Count™